Mind Your Weight

Mind Your Weight

By Deepak Rana

Neepradaka Press

Published by Neepradaka Press 2010
All rights reserved.

ISBN 978-0-9564928-1-4

Acknowledgements

A big thank you to all those that tried out the tools in this book and gave me your feedback. Without you this book would not have been possible.

Thanks to my publishers for supporting my very long book writing process.

Thanks to Deepti

Rest in peace Teana, Thomnus, Keana, Snoopy and Kingu

Also by Deepak Rana

The Secret Power of Lists

Beyond Cosmic Ordering

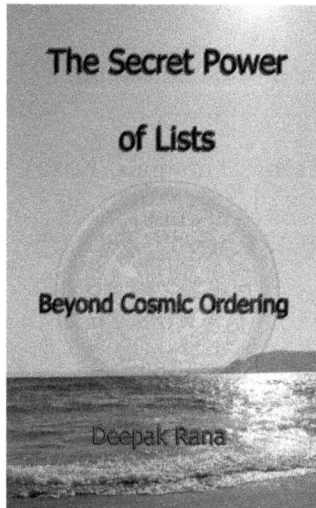

The Secret Power

of Lists

Beyond Cosmic Ordering

Deepak Rana

Listpower.mrdee.net

Mind Your Weight
Audio CD

Using advanced brain/mind technology

Discount details see back of book

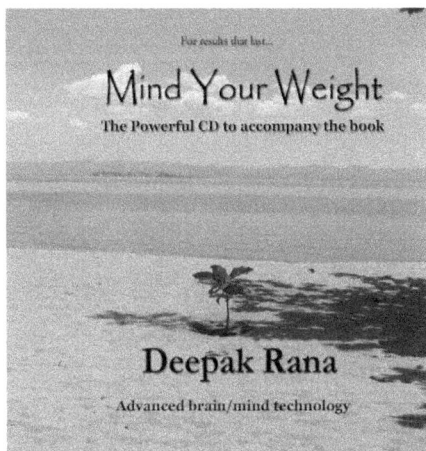

MindyourWeight.mrdee.net

Contents

Preface

This book follows on from the success of my first book 'The Secret Power of Lists', [1] I had a great deal of messages requesting further lists to help with other problems, as well as some additional advice and guidance.   One of the most common requests was about subjects dealing with weight problems.   These including problems with gaining weight, diet, exercise, binge eating, cravings and habitual eating.   I then began some research looking in to these problems and how they could be overcome using the Secret Power of Lists, as well other tools.   I soon had a couple of chapters completed of this book which was then sent out to a selection of people to read, and try out.   A couple of redrafts later, I had what I believe is the only guide you will ever need to lose weight and stay healthy.

Advanced Sound Technology CD

In the course of my research I was able to develop a powerful CD which includes scientifically based audio engineering, [2] coupled with a variety of other sound scripts.   The CD works by guiding the brain through various frequencies to tap deep in to the mind, and bring about change that would only be possible to advanced yogi's after years of mental training. [2]
There is a full guide at the back of the book, on how

to use the CD with the chapters of this book. You will also find a special coupon offering details about purchasing the CD at a discount.

Introduction

Many people are struggling with food and weight, and most will have been struggling since a young age. For example, Leena had been struggling for over 27 years to overcome her weight issues. It began from the time she saw herself as being fat, which caused her to decide not to take part in the many adventures of life. Looking back she said she wasn't actually overweight at the time. But the seed had been sown in her mind that she was fat. It caused her to make certain decisions in life. The side-effects actually led her to gain weight, and in other words she became her thoughts. It made her chronically unhappy and she believed that being fat was the main cause of her unhappiness. Leena, as do many people, went on a variety of

> I do the very best I know how-the very best I can; I mean to keep on doing so until the end.
> Abraham Lincoln

diets. Some of the starvation diets did seem to work for a short time, but within a month she would see her weight return. It seemed a lot of the diets worked for others but not for her, and she couldn't understand why. What she failed to understand was that the root cause was not the fat itself, and therefore attempts at getting rid of her fat would lead to failure.

You can read more about her story at the end of this chapter.

As I mentioned in my first book, the mind is a most powerful tool which can bring us the joys of life or pull us down in to the depths of despair. Our minds can be one of the main reasons that lead us to become overweight, and the main reasons why diets eventually fail. If we don't tackle the problems with the mind, we cannot make lasting progress with diets. The most successful health centers offering weight loss plans have been successful because they have taken in to account not just the body, but the mind as the focus of their efforts. Unfortunately such success has also meant increasing subscription costs, that are far out of the reach of many people. However you can get the same sort of success by using this book.

Those who do not suffer from any issues with weight may think it is a simple matter of eating less food and exercising more. Moreover, such people may comment that overweight people must be lazy. I believe this notion is incorrect. It assumes that it is an easy matter to 'eat less food', and that lack of exercise is just down to 'idleness'.

Consuming food is not always a conscious activity. This may be quite a surprising statement. How can someone not know they are eating? Well consider the act of driving. Every driver will have had the experience of driving along a familiar journey and surprised at having reached the end of the journey with no conscious recollection of having got there[3]. For some, this is the way it is with food. They will have opened a packet of snack, one after another with no conscious recollection of having done so. It is only after, when they look at the number of empty packets accumulated, that they are surprised at how much they have

> All our dreams can come true, if we have the courage to pursue them.
>
> **Walt Disney**

eaten. Some TV shows[4], trying to help people to look at their eating habits, have displayed on a table all of the food an individual has consumed during the week. Seeing it all on the table, that person is very surprised and shocked at how much they really have put in to their bodies. What is at play here is the subconscious compulsion to eat more food than is needed, and to stay indoors on the sofa doing nothing. Again, this book will tackle this issue.

As I said in the preface, I hope this is the last ever book you read on weight loss and that the tools provided will assist you throughout your life to stay at your healthy weight and have a healthy relationship with food. You may also find my first book a great deal of help in getting the other things you may want in life such as a new job, a new partner, or to increase the flow of money coming towards you.

The Power of the Mind

The Bhagavad Gita states that 'the mind acts like an enemy to those who do not control it'. This is especially true with regard to people with weight problems, as it is their minds which are actually their greatest enemy, and not the food on their plates. What I want to put across is that there are reasons for your weight and those reasons are rooted within the mind. If we can begin to tackle the mind, to control it, we can make it our friend rather than an enemy.

This book will bring you the tools to accomplish this and makes use of the Secret Power of Lists, as well as some other tools and techniques that came out of my research.

How long before I see results?

When I provided the first drafts of the book to a few people I was asked how long the process would take before they started to lose weight. Many assumed this was like one of the diets they had tried before which promised weight loss in 30 days and that would be the end of it.

My answer to them was that the process would be for a lifetime because the mind is always with us and does not go on holiday after 30 days. However the trial group did find that after a few months, they started to see small weight and other changes occurring within them, and were eager to continue using the tools provided in this book. I advised them to revisit the book every few months just to make sure that their mind was working as they wanted it, and to ensure the weight loss was a long lasting one.

For many people, they will be tackling a lot of deep rooted issues within the mind which will take time to overcome. But with this book you will overcome them. Furthermore, there may be times when the circumstances of life cause recurrent problems with weight, such as for example the shock from the death of a loved one. Again you will be able to use this book to help you cope, and make sure you overcome any associated problems. So do not think in the short term, but think long term. In the short term you may see the small changes in weight loss as not very significant, but seen over five years, all those small changes add up to a lot.

How to use this book

You may want to look at the contents page and browse through any topic of interest. However I would advise you to also read the other chapters, as it may be contain relevant information about something you may not have thought of. The other issue is that your mind may be subconsciously guiding you away from a particular chapter because it wishes for you to avoid change.

Observe any feelings you get when you gaze down the list of chapter titles, and notice whether you feel any tension or aversion around a particular title. This may be a clue that this chapter is of particular interest for you. If you wish to understand further why your mind may be subconsciously guiding you away from a chapter, then you may wish to read the explanatory introduction from 'The Secret Power of Lists'.

There is also a suggested introductory program at the back of the book which will take you through all the chapters in 3 steps. It has been designed to build upon the previous step so that you develop and grow as a natural progession. This is a useful program if you just don't know where to start, or if you want to avoid your subconcious from preventing you from reading a particular chapter.

<u>Do it</u>

All change must begin with action. So whichever chapter you read, the first, last or every chapter, make sure you take action. Do not allow yourself to put it off for another day. Take the decision now as you read this that you will take action as soon as you have finished reading a chapter. If you take no action from reading this book, then you have made a decision to allow yourself to be affected by what goes on around you, and are a slave to your mind. So why not take a decision to have full control of your mind, and of your life? We all have read about people who have led exceptional lives and overcome all kinds of odds to succeed. These people took the decision not to allow anything to effect what they wanted in life. So I urge you now to take the decision to take action.

Leena's Story

Leena

When I was young I developed a little faster than other girls, and so I was labelled incorrectly as being big and fat. I was neither of these and nor was I overweight. However the label got stuck and I started to believe I was big and fat. I really loved sports but other children's comments put me off it and I began to really dread any kind of sport. If I could use any excuse to avoid it, I would. So I would fake illness or injury whenever I could, and would sit on the bench's watching the other children take part in physical activity. School life was, in general, quite a sad time for me and I could never talk about it to my parents as I didn't want them to feel sorry for me. So at the dinner table when I was asked how school went, I would answer with one word, and then stuff lots of food in my mouth, so I wouldn't have to say anymore. This continued in to my teenage years and whenever anyone took interest in me I had a worry they would realise the truth that I was fat, and so I would always carry food around with me. So, to prevent anyone asking questions I would always be eating something so I looked to be 'too busy', and people would, I thought, not bother talking to me. As a result I put on lots of weight and became the fat person that I believed I was.

Chart Your Hunger

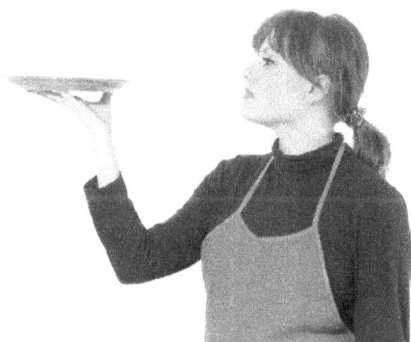

D o you eat when you are hungry?
D o you eat when your stomach is empty?

These two questions look the same but they are not. The feeling of hunger is not just a physical, but also a mental entity. You may feel as if you are hungry yet your stomach may not be empty. You may see a great visual feast before you, and after you have consumed so much of it, the visual appeal maybe such that you still feel a hunger. This is mental hunger.

Sometimes we are slaves to time which dictate that one must eat at specific times of the day and often we will eat plenty beforehand almost as if something is going to prevent us from eating at our specific time. This may be because we feel that if we don't eat beforehand we may overeat later. In others words, we are overeating beforehand in order to prevent possible overheating later. This can be something that can turn in to a lifetime habit, and what invariably happens is you will consume more than what the body needs, with the excess becoming fat. There has been lots of advice suggesting that eating a few small meals through the day will help with weight loss. The idea being that having small meals spread out will reduce the need to overeat at any time. However research has shown that the frequency of meals has no impact on weight loss, whether its three or more meals in the day$_6$. In other words, you could still be unknowingly overeating even if its spread out in small amounts in the day, or consumed in one or two sittings.

Many have forgotten what the signal is for hunger. The reason is that food not only serves a nutritional need, but also serves as an emotional satisfier. In other words, it satisfies some emotional needs that are connected with foods. It is what is termed by many as 'emotional eating'$_7$. These connections will begin in childhood where for example, sweets may have been put in to our hands when what we really needed was a hug. So when in times of emotional need we may turn to food, and this in turn becomes a repetitive behavior and becomes a habit. Once something becomes a habit it becomes an easy thing to do, as the mind does not need to think anymore, of how to deal with a lack of something, and instead will become preprogrammed to reach for its readymade solution. This will mean that over time you will have forgotten what the signals are for hunger, and instead, rely on your mind to tell you when (and what), to eat rather than your body. Another aspect to this, is that when we were young and experienced hunger pains, we may have had both hugs and food. The taking away of pain thus associated with hugs and food. In later life when we need a hug to heal a pain, and when a hug is not available, we will resort to a food substitute instead.

There are also associations of food with power and control. For example, what would be the result of a family which was not very loving, and the children were only given attention at mealtimes? Well, this may have resulted in a lot of tantrums by a child refusing to eat and leading to mom or dad paying a lot of attention to the child to make them eat. On the other hand it may be that the family was very controlling during the teenage years over all aspects of that child's life, and by not eating, allowed the child to feel they had some control over something. Chapter 3 deals with exploring your childhood food associations and how these can be broken.

But let us go back to the two questions at the start of the chapter, the first, do you eat when you are hungry, and the second, do you know when your stomach is empty. The next exercise will help you get started with charting your hunger. This will help you to understand where you are and then decide on whether to eat or not.

It will, over time, help you to understand your body and your mind, when making decisions on eating.

Action: Chart your hunger

Make several copies of the Hunger Chart in different sizes, and put them around several locations. For example, stick them on your fridge, cupboards, or your desk. carry a smaller version in your pocket or purse. Whenever you need to make a decision over eating, look at the chart, and begin by focusing your mind on your hunger and deciding at what level you are and whether you should decide to eat or not. The more you continue with the charting, the more proficient you will get with recognizing whether you are truly hungry.

The Hunger Chart

1	2	3	4	5	6	7	8	9	10
Feel painfully full	Very Full Slight pain	Full Can't eat more	Full but could eat bit more	Satisfactorily full	Not Hungry feel ok	Slight empty feeling	Distracted by hunger thoughts	Very hungry irritated slight pain	Extremely Hungry- no energy
Don't eat	Don't eat	Don't eat	Don't eat	Don't eat	Don't eat	Small snack	Eat	Eat	Eat

Food Associations

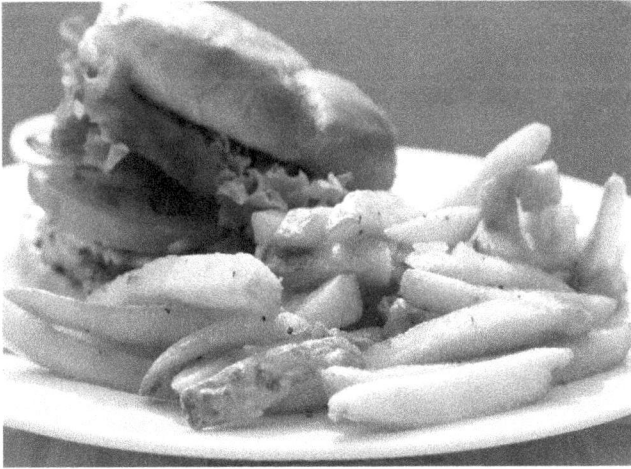

The previous chapter touched upon the subject of food and associations. Food has a strong emotional connection to us from the day we suck on a nipple. Such connections can be helpful or unhelpful depending on how we develop and grow, and the kind of life experience we have. Therefore it is important you examine what your own personal associations are with various types of foods, and the exercise described shortly will help. Have a read of the experiences of people who did the excercise (end of the chapter), to give you an idea about what the excercise aims to do.

The exercise

The following exercise will assist with looking at your own personal associations with food. This is a very powerful technique and so read through it all before you start, and cover as many years as you want during that session. Spend half a day during the week for a session, as you may find that any more than two sessions in the week may drain you both physically and mentally. Spread out over a couple of months will yield results. The feedback I have received has been that most have gained a lot from doing around three half day sessions in total over three weeks.

You will need the record sheet on the next page for each year of your life. Most will find that covering years 1 to 18 will be sufficient, as these are the most crucial years in your early development.

Food Association Record Sheet				
Age				
General Notes				
Memories of food- incidents/emotions				

Emotion Word Grid (Emo-word)

PAIN	JOY	ECSTACY	CONFIDENT	WEAK	TEMPER	CLEVER	TEARS
JUICY	ACRID	DECAY	WORRY	DISGUST	HONOUR	SMILE	CARE
PUNISHED	REPULSE	DEPRESSED	FRAGRANT	TASTY	BRIGHT	BROKEN	JEALOUSY
HAPPY	DENSE	CHEERFUL	DEFIANT	ANGER	SWEET	CLOSED	BLESSED
TART	DARK	WONDER	AROUSED	POSITIVE	SPARKLE	SOUR	LAUGHTER
TENSE	DELIGHT	CRABBY	POWERFUL	CHOKED	TWITCH	EXPOSED	CLUMSY
VALUED	DREAMY	BITTER	DESPAIR	DELIGHT	TENDER	HOPELESS	DESPISED
SULKY	SHIVER	NUMB	POWERLESS	COMFORT	FOUL	CREAMY	BLISS

Mind Induction

Begin with the following general relaxation to prepare your mind and body. This can be carried out sitting or whilst lying down. Some people will feel very sleepy when lying down, so may prefer to sit in a comfortable chair.

Loosen any tight clothing and take off your shoes if you are wearing them. Focus your attention on your breath until your breathing begins to slow and deepen. Keep your mind focused on your breath and try and visualise a peaceful image.

Begin to now focus attention to your feet, beginning at the toes. Starting with the toes, wiggle them to release any tension. Now rotate the ankles, and flex them. Move your attention to the calves and the long muscles of the thighs, and tense and relax them until you can let the tension go.

Now move your attention to your stomach and lower body. Tighten your stomach muscles and hold the tension for a count of five, and then release. Do this two more times, releasing tension each time you relax.

Now your shoulders and arms. Shrug your shoulders, tense and release your arms, then clench and release your hands. Do this three times and finally, release all tension and let your arms and shoulders relax.

Focus now on your facial muscles, opening the mouth and eyes wide three times and then consciously release tension and let your face relax. If you feel tension in your neck, turn your head slowly to the right and then the left a few times to allow the nect to relax. Finally, shift your attention to the very top of your head. Consciously tighten the scalp by lifting your eyebrows and then scrunching them.

Now with your body fully relaxed focus again on your breathing. Slowly draw in your breath to capacity then hold it for a count of 10. Then, slowly exhale your breath. Repeat this 5 times and then go on to the next exercise.

Focus your mind back to when you were at the age you have decided upon. Think about how you saw the world, think about the people you were with and then try and think about the food you will have eaten and where you were. You may feel you can't remember anything at all. This is normal, the main point is that you try and get the mind to at least focus in the past to that age. Whether you consciously remember anything, or not. Once you feel you have got as much as you can (allow at least ten minutes), get up and fill in your sheet. Do not delay the filling out of the sheet. There is space to make any general notes as well as any notes relating to food. Just write whatever comes to mind and try not to pre-analyse anything.

Now have a look at the emo-word grid and gaze at the grid for a few seconds. Look back at your notes and read them and then look at the grid and circle six words.

You will now have six words associated with foods that you can relate to a particular year of your life. You also will have the notes to provide you with a starting point for further investigation.

This you may wish to follow up by tracing an event during a particular year. Or you may wish to question people around you (parents, siblings), during that year, and if they have any recollections of events or issues around that time. This exercise's main purpose is to bring up associations so that the next step can be effective.

It doesn't matter if you feel nothing has come out from the exercise as it may be that your mind is blocking attempts at recall.

The next step-break through the association

The next step will use the Secret Power of Lists to help break through unhelpful associations with food.

Photocopy the grid on the next page, and fill the grid with the words you circled from the earlier exercise and the foods that you made notes of. The relevant boxes are labelled. Complete 6 sheets. Now with the first sheet scrunch it up and in your mind say 'I am letting you go'. Do the same with the other sheets. Then take the sheets and find somewhere far away from home to dispose of it. It is important that you do not keep the sheets at home after they have been filled in.

Breaking Food Associations: Grid

Emo-word	Food	Food
Food	Emo-word	Food
Food	Food	Emo-word
Emo-word	Food	Food
Food	Emo-word	Emo-word

Feedback

John

I decided to start at age 2, even though I couldn't consciously ever remember being two!

I made sure I was relaxed on my bed and made sure I would not be disturbed for at least a few hours. Closing my mind I tried to think as far back as I could to when I was a child. Soon I was getting various images in my mind, my mother, the trees around our house. I must have been about 5 at the time. I then tried to go further back and at first my mind just drew a blank, no images or anything. However I had feelings of being enveloped but I couldn't quite figure out what it meant. A few more minutes of this feeling and then I had a taste of a watery biscuit in my mouth along with a feeling. This was then mixed in with a feeling of being enveloped followed by watery biscuit. I then ended the exercise and filled in the sheets. Looking at it I realized that I had developed some kind of association with biscuits and being enveloped or suffocated. I realized that this actually explained why I tended to eat packets of biscuits dipped in tea whenever I was under a strain or in danger of being enveloped by events around me. It's not something I had been consciously aware of but actually my drawers at work have a big supply of these biscuits as well as drawers of them at home. I realized I had purchased so many because I had associated them with being enveloped and they were for me solution to times when I was in mental stress. I was able to ask my mother about biscuits and she told me that my father used to work in a biscuit rusk factory and used to bring home free broken biscuits which she would soften in water and feed me.

Anita

I didn't think I would get much out of the exercise as I didn't feel my childhood had any hidden skeletons. But I realized this exercise isn't supposed to be about revealing hidden secrets. The main aim was to bring to the surface food associations we all personally have. My friend may associate cakes with comfort and joy while another may associate cakes with something else. That was the case for me. Doing the exercise brought to the surface my association with cakes and being busy. I was always a creative child and my parents celebrated every single birthday and all I remember is always being busy a few days before my birthday as well as on the day. My parents would involve me with doing cards, or trying to blow balloons or making decorations. So my primary association with cake was being busy. It is very true that whenever

I'm busy with a project I'll buy cakes for when I'm too busy for a meal. What this exercise did was provide an understanding of the association and although it may not totally stop me buying cakes, at least I will be able to stop and think about it rather than unconsciously buying cakes. I haven't tried the next exercise to break associations- but hope to try that out very soon.

<u>Paul</u>

I tried the first two times to do the exercise lying on my bed. However I found that I must have been in need of proper rest because I fell asleep every time. I realised this was because I had been trying to do the exercise after I had come home from work. Normally I would be drinking coffee after work, have a large meal and lay on the sofa and then I would always wake up the next day with a struggle. But I found that in those two days when I had done the relaxation and fallen asleep, even though I had awoken late evening and had my meal, I was waking up more refreshed. So I realised just by doing the relaxation was of great benefit to me.

So I experimented with trying to do the exercise sat in a chair, and this worked for me. I didn't fall asleep and I still got the full benefit of the relaxation so the next morning I was feeling more refreshed than I had ever been. I also thought that maybe the phrase that I often used of me not being a 'morning person' was incorrect. Perhaps there is no such thing and the people who do feel they are not 'morning people' just haven't fully allowed their mind and body to rest?

About the exercise itself I was able to discover that I had a deep connection to my father and with cakes. My father had died when I was five years old and I didn't actually remember anything much about him. However doing the exercise I did get a few images of him and I had memories of people talking about my father in the past tense and my mother in tears, holding me close to her. I remember seeing a long table with various foods on and in particular I remember cup cakes in various colours, all with red cherries on top. I was given these cup cakes by various people and I therefore discovered that my connection to my father was related to these cakes. The wake therefore imprinted in me my mothers and everyone else's memories of my father with these cakes. Although it's the cupcakes I remember, there must have been other sweet edibles I must have eaten and they had association with my father.

Diet Plans

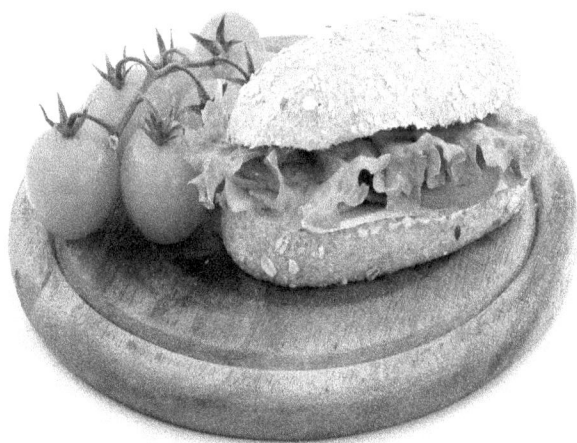

How many diet plans to lose weight have you undertaken in your life? If you have ever started one plan, then it is likely you will have started many others. Retail bookshelves are full of a various diet plans from the low-carb diet$_8$ to raw food diets. Why is it that there are so many diets, and why will they have worked for one person, but not for you? Well, everyone's mind is different, as are people's bodies. It is a combination of differences which explains why the same diet may work for those whose bodies are totally different, and also why a particular diet may fail for two bodies which are the quite similar. Then, how does one succeed with a diet plan? For a diet plan to succeed, it must be the right diet for you, and secondly your mind must be sufficiently prepared for success. If the mind is prepared, than you will find that a lot more of the variety of diets out there will bring you success, where in the past the same diets had brought disappointment.

<u>Choosing the right diet for you</u>

I would suggest that you start with a diet that will bring you the least difficulties. By this I mean difficulties with obtaining and preparing the items, as well as issues with your personal likes and dislikes. Also seek advice of your physician on healthy eating.

You may find that a simple healthy eating plan along with the mind techniques is all that you will need to start down the road of losing weight.

The following questions you should ask yourself when deciding on a diet plan:

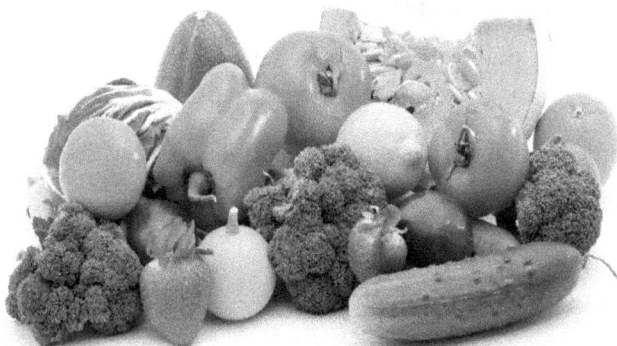

- Can you attend diet meetings on a regular basis?
- Do you like to cook or will you want something that is ready made?
- Do you gain a lot from working in a supportive group?
- Do you enjoy cooking and trying out new recipes?
- Do you have a small or large budget to spend on specialist items?

Listen to your body

You will find that as you progress with some of the exercises in this book, that you will also free the body to tell you what it truly needs for a healthy diet. There was some research carried out in the 1970's where children were allowed to pick whatever they wanted to eat for the month. Now these were young children, and when young we are much more in tune with our bodies and have yet to allow 'life' to take us down various twists and turns. The result was that these children made choices which, on examination, revealed that the foods chosen were what we would consider to be a suitable balanced diet for a human being. If you read through chapter 4 you will find an exercise to do with reconnecting to the child you were all those many years ago. This will assist with learning to listen to your body and to develop positive feelings towards healthy foods.

Water

Do not neglect the importance of drinking water[9]. Consider that a large percentage of your body is water, and a lot of your bodily processes need water for their proper optimum function.   In some cases the craving for foods can be the result of the body needing water. If in the past your body's need for water has been via food then you will crave foods when it requires water. You can slowly break your body's need for food by feeding it what it really needs: water. One quick and easy test to check if your body is in need of water is to observe the colour of your urine. It should be of a light colour. Any darker means you need to take some water. You may also want to consider the quality of the water you drink. It is common practice for some countries to add fluoride as well as other chemicals to tap water for its benefits. Although such benefits in comparison to possible risks is still debated. There are also other considerations with regard to tap water such as the chemicals added during treatment of the water and the pipework the water has had to travel through to get to your tap[9]. The choice is yours whether to continue drinking the water, as it may be that there are extremely low levels of contaminants in your tap water. You can arrange to have your water tested for any contaminants, and you may then wish to use filters on your tap water to eliminate any particular contaminants identified. A filter may well be the best choice in comparison to the cost of purchasing bottled spring water for your needs.

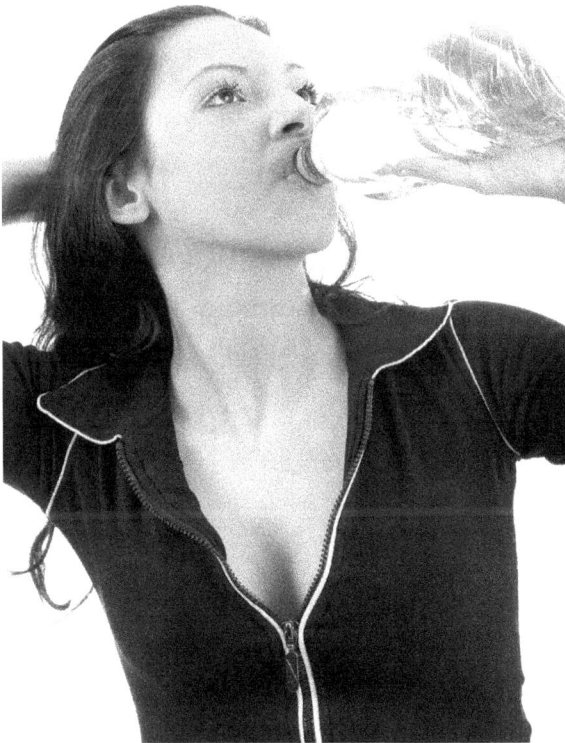

So let us begin looking at the mind preparation techniques to assist with diet plan success.

<u>Energising and de-energizing foods</u>

The processes here will allow you to prepare your mind to develop a fondness for some foods and aversions to others. Although this will not cause you to completely avoid certain foods, it will program your mind to crave them less and less. For those healthy foods which you may have a slight dislike of, or have a neutral feeling towards, the processes here will help you to choose them more readily than other options. For example, when entering a restaurant you will gravitate towards healthy salad options and feel indifference or an aversion to the cream cakes. Or when shopping, you will feel more drawn towards some food options than others. The processes described are very powerful and I have had a lot of positive reports from them. To quote a one example, one email I received from a lady in the UK whose main problem was consumption of ready meals. She states 'for the past 10 years I have been continually buying ready meals. At the start this was because I had no time to cook with a new job, but then after a promotion I found I had time on my hands in the evening. But I still purchased ready meals as I felt lazy to cook, and when I did attempt to cook I found it tasteless compared to my ready meals. This was not healthy and I was very overweight. I started exercise which helped a little but I knew my main problem was these ready meals. I started energizing some vegetables and de-energising ready meals. One night in the supermarket I passed by some vegetables and they just seemed so colourful and popped out at me. So I purchased a whole lot of them. It was the first time I had walked past the ready meals section without buying any. At home I couldn't wait to try the veggies so I just quickly steamed them. What was strange is that I ate them without any flavouring and they felt so juicy and tasty in my mouth I couldn't get enough of them. I haven't totally got rid of my ready meal addiction but I'm eating them maybe once or twice a week and the other times I'm trying out lots of different vegetables. I feel a lot better in myself and feel I am finally going to have success with losing weight'.

The Exercise

The two processes that follow should not be done together. Complete one process and then begin the other. So for example you can conduct the energising process for the minimum of a week followed by a week of the de-energising process. You cannot however do an energising process for 2 days and then start the de-energising process the next day.

The energising process

Use this process to energize any food. The most common things are vegetables. I would suggest getting a small bowl and fill it with samples of vegetables of different types. Next you will need a large piece of paper, and begin writing out the list of Sanskrit words in the first column shown on the next page. I have provided an English translation as well as a transliteration of the page. It is important to read the words as you write them. Details of the importance of reading them out loud is described in my book 'the secret power of lists' which talks about sound vibration and its effects.

Once the list is complete place the bowl on top of the list for 24 hours, after which you can then make use of the vegetables in your cooking. You should continue to do this for at least a week, and no longer than a month. This will create strong positive connections to the particular foods used during the process (in this case vegetables).

Sanskrit	Translation	Transliteration
शक्ति	Energy	Zakti
देह	Body	Deha
निरामय	Health	Niraamaya
उद्धार	Repair	Udhaara
स्तास्नु	Stable	Staasnu
तेजते	Energise	Tejate

De-energising food

You may have seen the 'Paris in the the Spring' illusion where the words are put in a triangle. Most people will find that they fail to see the extra word that is printed. The mind has masked it out because it has seen it and recognized it as not important to complete the sentence. Similarly when you walk past a de-energised item in the supermarket your mind may well not 'see' them and you will walk right past them. So lets get on with the de-energising process.

This is a process to de-energise food for which you are trying to cut down on or avoid. It will cause your mind to avoid them at restaurant either by actively making you feel an aversion or by masking them from your vision. By this I mean the same kind of masking that sometimes goes on when we fail to see something which is right in front of us. For example have you ever been tense about a particular trip and failed to find your car keys. Then, someone else will point the keys out to you which have been right in front of your eyes but you had failed to see them. Your subconscious mind had masked the keys from your vision. This can also work in the reverse whereby if you have been looking to buy a particular make and colour car, you then start to see that colour and make of car wherever you go, and wonder where they have all come from. In fact they had been there all the time, but now your subconscious had a reason to focus on them and pick them out.

So let us begin with de-energising process. Enter a relaxed state of mind by using the mind induction in Chapter 2. Once your mind and body is relaxed, I want you to imagine a table with plates of the various foods that you wish to de-energise. If there is only one food you want to de-energise then imagine a dozen plates all with the same food on it. Try and imagine the foods in as much detail as possible. Look at the colours and smells and touch them to feel the texture.

Now I want you to think back to when you were physically sick from an upset stomach. I want you to imagine that feeling of sickness and keep it with you as you continue to look at the foods on the table. Now feel that sense of sickness get from bad to worse on an ever sliding scale. Once you can not stand the feeling of sickness any longer, I want you to push the plates off the table until they come crashing to the floor. As each plate falls off the table I want you to feel your sickness reducing as each plate falls. When the last plate has come off the table I want you to feel a sense of calm and joy. Bask in this calm for a few minutes and then you may get up.

Some items useful for diets

I did not want to offer any recipes in this book and wanted to let the reader use my advice to select the right diet for them. But what I do provide on the next few pages are some items which you may wish to use within your diet pans.

Red Bush Tea

This is something I have been recommending people drink instead of tea or coffee as their morning drink.

Redbush or rooibos grows in the Western Cape Province of South Africa. The tea is harvested from the leaves which turn red when they have been fermented. I have drunk this tea for many years and it has for me a sweet mellow taste that is unmatched by any drink I have had before. I also find that I use very little sugar due to the natural sweet taste of the tea.

Redbush tea has been found to contain the following minerals: iron, potassium, magnesium, zinc, calcium and sodium, as well as a particular flavonoid. Unlike tea and coffee Red Bush tea contains no caffeine, and has a very low tannin content. Tannin can have a few negative effects which can be discovered for yourself by consulting other health books.

Tulsi

This plant is also called Holy Basil (Ocimum tenuiflorum) It has been a widely used plant in India for thousands of years for both religious and medicinal purposes. It's extracts are used for various remedies ranging from cough, colds, heart disease, inflammation and much more. The reason I include this plant here is that it can be used for making tea as a general tonic. It is quite difficult to raise the tulsi plant from seed so I would suggest you obtain a cutting from an existing plant from which it is quite easy to root and grow in to a new plant. Tulsi likes warm weather and enough water so that the top soil does not feel dry to the touch. You can pick the leaves once you have a large enough plant so there are still enough leaves for the tulsi to stay alive and grow. Apart from the general drink tonic, you can chew the leaves for coughs, sore throat or for various other conditions. The tea can also be used as hair shampoo or to put on the skin to help with any skin conditions. Contact me via the publishers at np@mrdee.net if you have difficulties obtaining this plant.

Honey

You may think at first that honey is sugary and therefore not good for you. The suggestion I give below will give you the benefits that honey provides, without worrying too much about excess sugar consumption. You will need to mix a spoon of honey with some juice from a fresh lemon in a glass of warm water. Drunk first time in the morning it will assist with providing you with both energy, as well as allowing the body to flush itself of toxins accumulating in the night, as well as during the day.

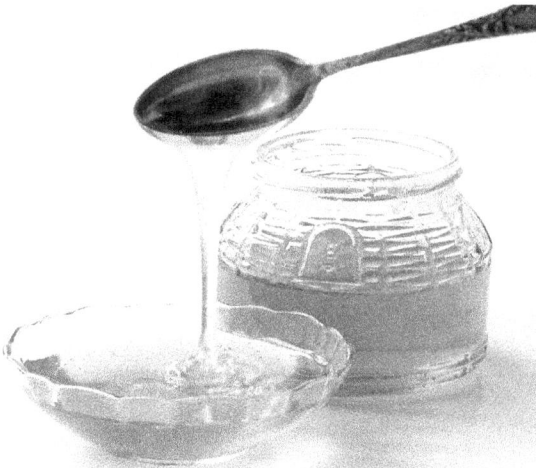

Feedback

Jo

Over the years I have tried almost every diet you can think of. The first diet started when I was very young, about 11 I think. Like all girls I wanted to be thought of as pretty and I was led to believe that being extremely thin meant I would be pretty. I was a little chubby and so I started my first ever diet. I basically watched everything I ate and tried to cut portions down to the minimum. It was difficult during meal times at home so I found sneaky ways to get less food on my plate. It didn't last long, as I would get really bad hunger pangs in the nights. More diets followed, and the pattern was the same. They all preceded from a particular event. Like a wedding to attend, or some party, or a holiday, where I needed to look my best. So I would start a diet and the diet varied depending on what magazine or books I had been reading. I can't say there was any diet that actually dramatically caused a great weight lost. I mean that although I had lost a little weight, it was not as dramatic as I wished. I always felt I could have done better, perhaps with a different diet.

How you see yourself

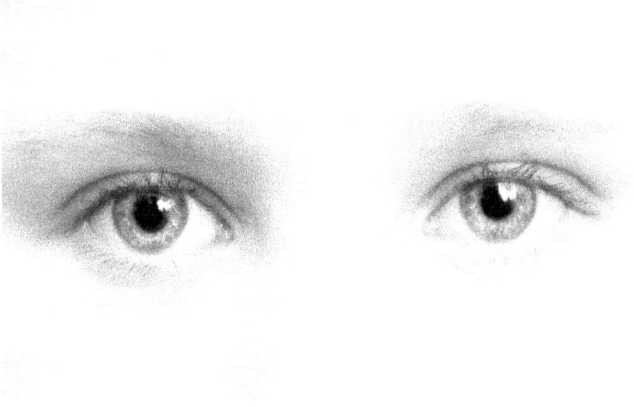

How you see yourself is an important question that you need to think about. The first step in looking at how you see yourself is knowing who you are. So what I would like you to do is take a piece of paper and write a very short statement about who you think you are.

Now compare that with the statements on the next page:

Who are you?

I'm 32, a housewife with five great kids

I'm 40, male, working as a business consultant with a lovely wife

I'm a positive person and work in publishing which reflects my personality

I'm 5 feet tall and, brown eyes and love painting

I'm a young lady who works as a care worker and vote liberal

I'm a bit of an overweight person, and weak when it comes to food

Was your statement similar to those? Did you mention an age, weight or occupation, or the number of children you have, or whether you were single or married? These are the kind of things you would tell someone that you have just met. By sharing these details we assume it has started us down the road of getting to know the other person better. Of course all things may be the facts of your life, and show your history in work and in life, the decisions you made and so on. But are they who you are?

I say they are not you- what is you is what causes inner stirrings of joy which reveals your true self. Now this could be a hobby or pastime, something in school that you loved to do, or a particular subject you love to read about and your ears prick up when the subject is mentioned. These loves are what makes you 'you'.

Now what does all this have to do with losing weight? Well when you are exploring your loves, whether it is painting or trying out guitar, you are allowing yourself to express your true self. As you allow your true self to expand and grow, you will become more in tune with your body and you will start to identify yourself in a positive manner. Instead of seeing yourself as fat and unattractive, you will see yourself as a valued human being capable of love, and being loved. It will provide impetus for you to seek out new ways of expressing yourself in the world. You will find that you don't need to jump start yourself out of bed every morning and drag yourself to work.

Have you wondered how it is that successful people seem to have boundless energy, and are able to wake up in the early hours, as if not to waste a minute more than necessary in sleep. How is it they are able to face their vocation in life with hundred percent enthusiasm every single day? It is because these people have explored their loves and found something they truly love to do and feels right for them. They have discovered something which they know within themselves they were meant to do. So how do you begin the process of discovering your joys? The process begins with going back to when you were a child and rediscovering your sense of exploration and play. When you found an interesting object as a child you did not go through a multitude of thoughts about whether you should reach for the object, or the consequences of doing so, or whether it would look good having the object in your hand. You simply reached out and grabbed the object. Now, if you were distracted and lost sight of the object did you go through days and days of regret over an object you never got to hold? No, you simply turned your attention to other interesting objects that came your way. However as you grew older and entered school you were no longer allowed the right to explore what you wanted. You were not given opportunities to fully explore those things which gave you pleasure. So if you happened to love mixing various paints you may well have been told to put the paints down, and do something more 'useful', like learn timetables. For some individuals, they may have still maintained their love of painting throughout childhood to later adult life and subsequently made it their life vocation. You may have read about successful people who remember the first stirrings of talent in early childhood, and how they continued to make use of these talents, even when discouraged to do so.

You can use the following exercise to focus your mind back to when you were a child and to rediscover some of the things you enjoyed doing which you may have forgotten about. This will allow you to reconnect to your true self. Use this as an impetus to explore further. For example if you discover a love of making things, why not join a club to try it out? You may discover you have a real talent and wish to grow further in this. There are some interesting stories at the end of the chapter of people who tried this exercise, and how they rediscovered their true selves.

Remembering your joys

U se the relaxation (mind induction) from Chapter 2. Once your body and mind is relaxed, focus your thoughts towards your childhood. Just explore whatever comes to mind, and let whatever images flow to you to come and go as they please. You may find that nothing comes to you at first. But continue doing this exercise everyday, and during those days observe any changes that occur within you. For example you may notice you are singing a lot, or you may be doodling a lot more than normal. Use all these as clues in discovering yourself. Read about some of the other peoples experiences in doing this exercise, to give you an idea of some of the things that may happen with you and what can come from your discoveries.

Feedback

<u>Diane</u>

From doing the exercise I was immediately getting images of school when I was a little girl and getting images of playing in sand. This I didn't think anything much about because nearly everyone will have the same memories of playing in sand. It was when I did the exercise a second time that I got memories of playing with plasticine. I loved making things from it. But in those days plasticine was not like it is today. The one we had in school was quite smelly and a bit oily, and I think at some point they must have totally stopped using them, as I don't have further memories of it. So after this exercise and pondering it some more, I thought I would do something silly and actually buy some plasticine. So I came home one afternoon with plasticine and I felt really silly getting this out on the table and playing about with it. After a couple of minutes of not doing much with it apart from squishing it and rolling it I started feeling quite relaxed and daydreamy. It's like the feeling you get sitting outside on a hot summers day. I started to make shapes and then I felt I wanted to make a head, so I did. I found some things in the kitchen to cut and shape it and I ended up with something I never thought I was capable of doing. I left that head on the mantelpiece and a friend had come round one day and asked me who did it, and commented it was quite good, and when I said I had done it, she was really surprised. You see I'm an accountant and deal with facts and figures, so not considered an 'arty' person. I went on to buy some real clay and I am now sculpting on my weekends. It's so meditative when I'm sculpting and its just helped with reducing work stress and I've rediscovered my sense of touch. There's a special feeling I get when I touch the clay with my hands.

Meena

My experience was really interesting. I have been married ten years, to a man who is a mechanical engineer. So there are always bits of metal around the house and I'm forever trying to tell my husband to keep his things in the garage. But he loves tinkering with anything mechanical when watching t.v., so he likes to keep them around him. Now I thought I had nothing in common with this aspect of my husband's life. But when I did the exercise I discovered that as a child I was the one who loved building things. So whether it was plastic bricks, or bits of wood I was always playing with them and trying to put things together to make things. I wondered maybe thats why

I was attracted to my husband when I had met him. Although I had thought it was the physical attraction that was the initial charge that got us together. So on discovering this I started to try and understand what my husband was doing when he was tinkering with various metal parts. To my surprise I started to enjoy learning about how things fitted together. My husband finds it strange that I have suddenly found this hidden interest, and our relationship has got much stronger.

Get Moving

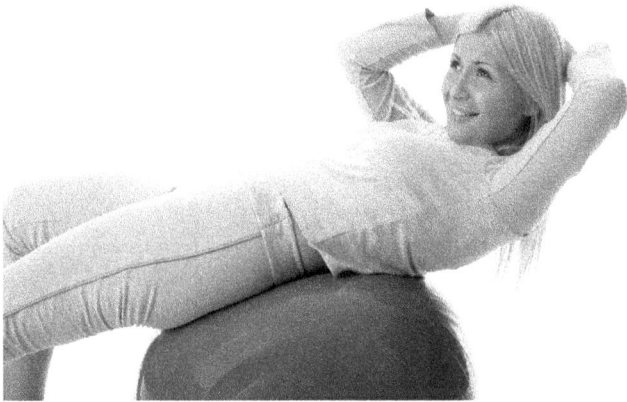

It may have been a long time since you have done some regular physical exercise. But diet and exercise must go hand in hand if you want to lose weight and stay fit. Exercise, apart from its physical benefits will also benefit your mind. Your ability to cope with stressful situations will improve as well as your ability to focus your mind with an acute sharpness.

This chapter will provide you with some mind techniques to get you from zero exercise to regular sustained exercise. The first step will be to get your mind motivated enough to start that very first exercise task. The second, and often the most difficult step, will be to maintain exercise on a regular basis. I have had many people tell me that they had started an exercise regime with such great determination, and were able to maintain it for a few weeks or months. But then the motivation level dropped and they exercised less and less, until they were back to square one[10]. Often these exercise sessions began at the start of the year after Christmas, when most people feel they have eaten too much and need to lose weight. Or they may have been given free gym subscriptions as Christmas gifts by a well meaning relative. Or, the sessions have begun when a beach holiday has been booked and they have wanted to ensure they looked good in beach wear.

Such people have told me of the pain of it all, both the physical and mental pain of exercising intensively for those few months. Plus the subsequent pain of not being able to maintain it for long or seeing very minor changes.

Now what if these same people were undergoing regular, but less intensive exercise throughout the year? There would be a lot less pressure and a lot less stress and the health benefits of feeling fit would stay with them throughout. So that is the focus of this chapter. To get your mind and body working as one to keep you gently exercising on a regular basis. I make the point here that it must be gentle exercise to start with. Even if you have previously worked out and feel you can push yourself harder I would urge you not to. The reason being that if you start exercising at high intensity, then at some point you will feel you cannot maintain it, you will cause your mind to want to steer away from exercising any more. By starting off with gentle exercise you will be able to maintain it, and your mind will not have any opportunity to associate the gentle exercise to pain. In fact by using the technique you will actually find yourself wanting to rush home to complete your exercise routine for the day. Over a long period of this gentle exercise you can, if you wish, add some intensive workouts- but always remembering to still maintain your gentle exercise sessions at all times. This way, even when you have a bad day, and don't feel like an intensive workout, you can still complete your daily gentle exercise session. There are only two exercises to do. So this is truly something you can follow for the rest of your life.

The Exercises

(1) Step on step off

This is a gentle exercise to get the leg muscles to move. The lower half of your body has a lot of muscles and more muscles working mean they need every bit of energy from your body in the form of calories.

Before I give you the exercise, let me first give you a mind exercise to go hand in hand with the physical exercise. Use chapter 2 for getting your body relaxed. Then focus on your heartbeat, feel the blood pumping through your body, feel the beat of the heart as it pumps. Now find a step and step one leg on as if climbing the step. Once both feet are on the step, step off. Now repeat, but with the other leg leading. As you do so recall the heartbeat exercise and step in rhythm to it. This will create a strong mind/body connection. This should be done 15 minutes each day.

<u>(2) Wall press-ups</u>

Repeat the body relaxation exercise from Chapter 2, but this time associate the heartbeat with pushing against the wall. Do this by stretching out both hands and place palms flat against the wall. Now bend the elbows so you bring your body close to the wall. Now breathe out as you push out on the first heartbeat and breath in as you feel the second beat, and lower yourself back towards the wall. It will take some time before you get in to the correct rhythm, so do not worry too much about getting it 'right'.

This should be done 15 minutes each day.

Feedback

Nikita

I go through periods where I will exercise and then stop. Anything can trigger these periods off. I might come across a book about health, and it provides me with some motivation to go out running or just exercising on the cross trainer thing I have at home. I will probably continue for about two weeks on a regular basis and then on the third week things would start to fall apart. The motivation would be gone and I would be back sitting on the sofa, and forgetting all about the exercise I had done the previous weeks. On the odd day I would probably try and get a little exercise done but then those days would be very rare until I was back to doing nothing at all.

Jonathan

It was quite clever the way there was only two exercises to do, and so I was feeling I could do this easily. I have a big problem with getting motivated with anything physical. After the first week I thought I was going to quit, but because the exercises had been so easy I had no reason to stop. Three weeks passed and I still was doing the exercises, and feel better in myself that each day I have used up some calories.

Feed the Mind

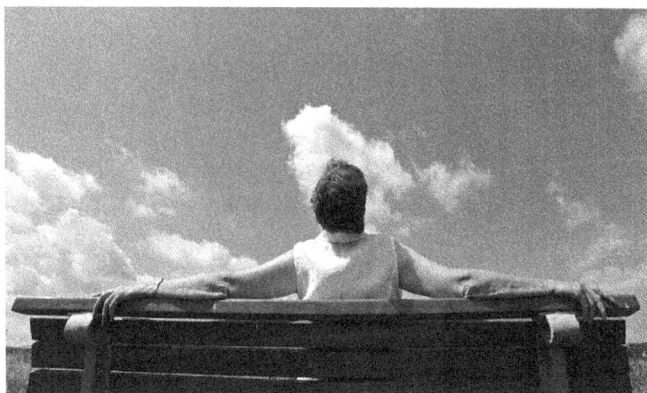

Meditation trains the
mind to be more
observant. Observing
the breath is a good start.

The mind, just as the body, needs to be fed a good quality diet. When the mind is fed with calmness it promotes bodily relaxation. This lowers the heart rate, and in turn unites the mind and body. You are more able to detach yourself from troubling thoughs.

Relaxation

I would urge you to try and spend at least a few minutes a day to relax and quieten the mind. There are many health benefits from relaxing the mind, and is used a lot in many therapies to heal the body. I will outline a very simple relaxation (meditation) technique here.

However if you wish to explore this further you can attend meditation classes either following Indian yogic disciplines or the Chinese tai chi.

Formal relaxation techniques

Begin by creating the right enviroment. This will depend on the space you have available to you. Try and find a quiet place, but be aware that you may not always be able to control some noise. However try and make it a comfortable and welcoming place and you will soon be able to filter out distracting noises. You may decide to sit on a mat or rug on the floor. Use cushions or blankets to make things comfortable. Or alternatively you can sit on a chair that has a sturdy back.

Relax the body

I am reproducing the body relaxation technique I introduced in chapter 2. It is a very powerful way of getting the body relaxed enough for the mind to operate at its best.

Focus your attention on your breath until your breathing begins to slow and deepen. Keep your mind focused on your breath and try and visualise a peaceful image.

Begin to now focus attention to your feet, beginning at the toes. Starting with the toes, wiggle them to release any tension. Now rotate the ankles, and flex them. Move your attention to the calves and the long muscles of the thighs, and tense and relax them until you can let the tension go. Now move your attention to your stomach and lower body. Tighten your stomach muscles and hold the tension for a count of five, and then release. Do this two more times, releasing tension each time you relax. You may find yourself adjusting the angle of your lower back as you encounter and release tension. Now your shoulders and arms. Shrug your shoulders, tense and release your arms, then clench and release your hands.   Do this three times and finally, release all tension and let your arms and shoulders relax.

Focus now on your facial muscles, opening the mouth and eyes wide three times and then consciously release tension and let your face relax. If you feel tension in your neck, turn your head slowly to the right and then the left a few times and finally, settle the neck to relax. Finally, shift your attention to the very top of your head. Consciously tighten the scalp by lifting your eyebrows and then scrunching them.

Now with your body fully relaxed focus again on your breathing. Slowly draw in your breath to capacity then hold it for a count of 10. Then, slowly exhale your breath. Repeat this 10 times, at which time you will enter a light meditative state. You can take yourself away to anywhere in the world. Why not take a trip to one of your favourite holiday destinations. I myself often take myself away to Rhodes in Greece where I am sat in the shade of a tree overlooking the light blue sea and feeling the cool air on my face. When I awake from my mediation I really feel as if I have been away.

Deeper Relaxation

If you wish to go in to deeper meditative states you may wish to visualise walking down a spiral staircase. Use as much of your senses to try and create the spiral staircase in your mind. As you walk further down the staircase, you will be able to enter a deep part of yourself. When you are ready you can walk back up the staircase.

> **Enlightenment is an experience that can happed as a result of meditation.**
>
> **Bhagavad Gita**

There are other indirect ways of relaxing the mind so seek out opportunities to do the following whenever you can, depending on your own interests. For example:

* Visit an art gallery
* Take a trip to peaceful natural surroundings- lake, park, beach.
* Sit in the garden and observe the plants, birds and insects.
* Do something creative like painting or a craft.

Sitting

I advocate sitting and doing nothing. You may wonder that simply sitting doing nothing is wasting time. But this is incorrect. Sitting doing nothing helps the mind to think better. Solutions to problems often come from sitting in a relaxed state. It is both refreshing and a very good use of your time. A great many celebrated thinkers knew the value of spending time doing nothing but sitting and daydreaming. Einstein for example would daydream a lot, and from these daydreams he was able to come up with breakthroughs in scientific thinking.

Mindful Awareness

What about when you are engaged in an activity? Is it possible to feed the mind at such times?

> **With Mindful Awareness you will be able to recall all those moments of life we tend to forget.**

Yes. The technique is called Mindful Awareness. This is simply taking the choice to fully notice what is happening in the moment. So if for example you are doing something ordinary such as making a cup of tea, do it with mindful awareness. To accomplish this, notice each aspect of the task. So for example notice the feel of the teabag as you place it in the cup. Listen to the sound of the water as it hits the cup. Notice the feel of the hot steam pass by your face and the smell of the tea as it brews. Mindful Awareness is also about taking your relaxed mind in to the outer world. Be aware and observant of the world around you as it happens. By becoming more observant and perceptive of your surroundings the more connectiveness you will feel with life itself.

Sleep

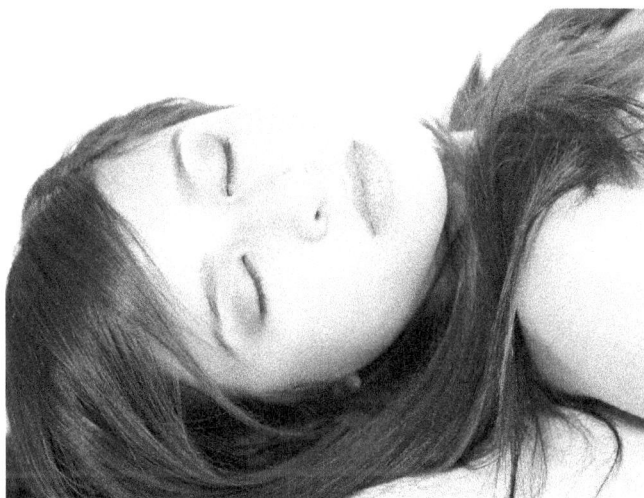

Sleep aids both the mind and the body, and it is essential you get good quality sleep. This means a full seven hour sleep period. Obviously some days you may sleep a few hours less, but as long as you maintain seven hours at least 5 days in the week you will benefit. Less sleep can cause all kinds of imbalances with your metabolism, and can lead to issue with diabetes, high blood pressure, memory loss, and weight gain. So take the decision to get an adequate amount good quality sleep.

There are some general agreed guidelines to aid restful sleep and these include:

• Sleeping by 11pm. A lot of bodily processes will begin after 11 and end a few hours later. By sleeping later you prevent the process from completing properly and has knock-on effects with other processes that follow on from it.

• Make sure your room is as comfortable for sleep as possible. This means as close to darkness as you can make it.

• Do not eat anything for at least an hour or two before your bedtime as this will prevent your body from wasting its energy on digesting foods

- Avoid all stimulants in the bedroom- this includes TV/radio and books. However peaceful reading materials and calming music is ok. You may wish to use my audio CD to feed your mind.

A lot of people suffer from not being able to get to sleep, or if they do, find they wake up in the middle of the night and cannot get back to sleep until early morning. There is a list in my previous book to help with this and I have included that here for you.

The list given in the next page or two, is reproduced from my first book on the secret power of lists. It will bring about a restful mind, which will aid peaceful sleep. So whether you have always had trouble sleeping, or whether it has become a recent problem, this list will help.

The list here calls for the use of a small piece of rose quartz. The stone will be able to harness the power of the list and aid restful sleep when placed under the pillow. Therefore find a piece that is small enough not to cause discomfort when placed under the pillow. Stones such as quartz are used extensively in India, placed in rings, or worn as jewellery. They are used mainly to aid in overcoming the negative aspects of certain planets, based upon an individuals particular astrological chart. But they can also be used in general for health benefits.

The List

Place a piece of paper in front of you and place the rose quartz at the top of the paper. Begin to write the sanskrit words in the first column on your peice of paper. You can write it across your paper. As you write, read the words in the third column which is a transliteration of the sanskrit. The middle column is just to show you what the words mean.

Now once you have written the words once, it will count as one set. Complete five sets in total making sure you speak the words slowly so the sounds vibrate within you and the quartz. Ths list is now complete.

Place the list under your pillow along with the piece of quartz. As a further aid to sleep you may read the list before going to bed. It is important for you to speak the words. Read the list as many times as you can before you feel sleepy.

You can continue with the list until peaceful sleep is restored. This should bring results in two months, and so if problems persist it may be worth looking at the other factors affecting sleep. These were touched upon at the beginning of the chapter.

> **We are such stuff as dreams are made on, and our little life is rounded with a sleep.**
>
> **William Shakespeare**

Sanskrit	Translation	Transliteration
शान्ति	Peaceful	Zaanti
रजानी	Night	Rajani
शान्त	Calm	Zaanta
शम	Restful	Zama

Emergencies

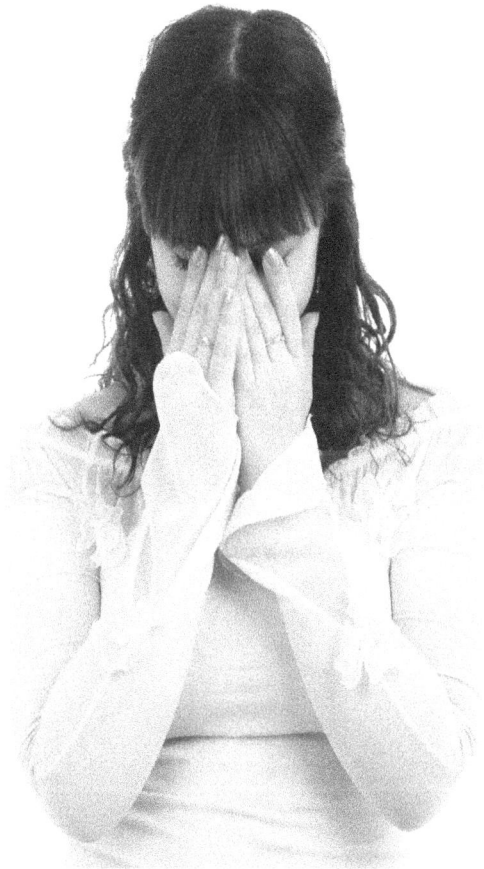

L ife does often throw emergencies at us which stops us right in our tracks and may even start to reverse progress made so far. Emergencies will often make you feel that you have no control over anything and you may start to consume everything you can and spiral in to a depression.

I will provide some useful tips and techniques here and will introduce you to two powerful lists that will help you through any emergency.

The first thing to know is that your ability to cope with any emergency is dependent on the foundations you have laid down. This means that everything in this book that you have made use of, will already have provided you with strong roots that will be the basis of your personal strength. Remember whatever the emergency is, you are not alone in having experienced it.

I will provide here a mediation tool that will allow your mind to remain calm and focused and settle down your nervous system resulting from the emergency. This is most common reason that mediation is prescribed as tool to help with stress.

When and where

It is Essential you find at least 30 minutes in the day to conduct the meditation. For many the best time is in the morning when the day has not yet begun and it will thus help set your mind up for the rest of the day. However any other time is suitable as long as you are uninterrupted. Find a place which is peaceful- this can be whichever room in the house you like, or it can even be an outdoor location. Many people for example find that sitting on the grass in the summer with the sounds of nature around them to be highly peaceful and soothing.

Now follow the relxation technique described in chapter 2.

Once relaxed do the following:

Imagine a very large open suitcase on your bed with nothing inside it. On the floor you have various clothes that you own and on each of them is a lable. These labels have words on and these words can be anything that you have worries or fears about, or can be emotions and feelings. For example, terror, despair, loneliness, death, spiders. Now pick up one peice of clothing at a time and look at the table you have attached to it. Now fold that peice of clothing and put it in the suitcase. Add as many more clothes as you want. Once you are finished, close the suitcase and zip it up. Now imagine taking that suitcase out of the house where there is a taxi waiting. You will open the door and put the suitcase in. Now tell the driver what you want to do with these fears, worries and emotions. You can be strong in your words such as 'get these damned fears out of my life'. Now watch the taxi drive away far away never to be seen again. Allow yourself a few moments to rest and then you may awake.

> **Keep calm, keep your mind clear, and do not be overcome by your fears.**

Suggested Introductory Programme

Here is a suggested programme to implement the tools provided in the book. This is a programme that will cover all aspects covered in this book and is done in three steps. It will introduce you to all topics covered in the book and each step will build upon the previous step. The diagram on the next page shows you what is included in each of the steps and the relevant chapter.

Step 1 prepares the body and mind for step 2 by offering relaxation techniques and ensuring your sleep is restful and beneficial. Two weeks is allowed for you to explore the excersises.

Step 2
This is the main part of the programme and 4 weeks is allowed to cover the topics. These will look deeper at your mind and body and issues with weight loss.

Step 3
This step is assisted by both step 1 and 2. You can now use the suggestions in the Diet plan, and look to start to get moving by using techniques in the Mind and Movement chapter.

Suggested Introductory Programme

Step 1	Step 2	Step 3
Feed the Mind (Ch.6)	How you see yourself (Ch.4)	Diet Plans (Ch.3)
Sleep (Ch.7)	Food Associations (Ch.2)	Get Moving (Ch.5)
	Chart your Hunger (Ch.1)	

Guide to using audio CD

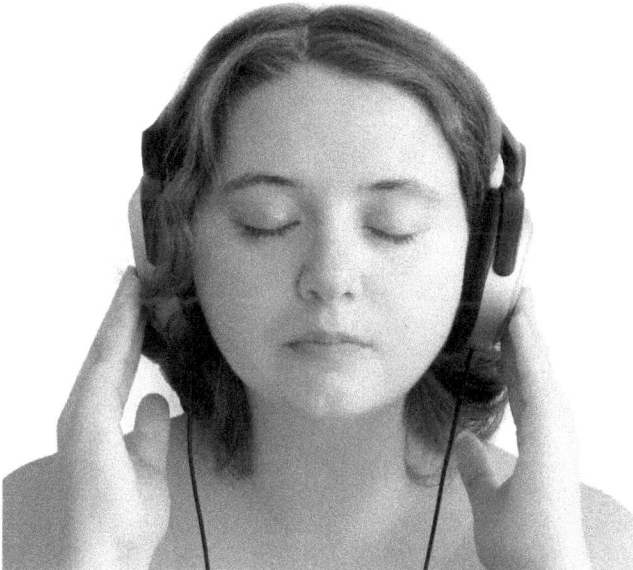

See the back page for details on obtaining the CD at a substantial discount.

Track 1: Entrance

This track should be used on a daily basis. It will help with your overall well being and peace of mind. The track also is beneficial in enhancing the effectiveness of other tracks. If you are new to sound technology then try using track 1 for a couple of days to get used to the feelings of relaxation.

Track 2: Discoverance

This track goes well with Chapter 4 which will guide your mind in to the theta state which is associated with dreams and fantasy.

Track 3: Hunger

An ideal track for Chapter 1. Will aid in developing a strong mind body connection so you can listen to your body's hunger signals.

Track 4: Food Associations
An aid to break your emotional connections to unhealthy foods.

Track 5: Sleep
It is best to make sure you are fully comfortable in your bed before you use this CD. If your mind is full of chatter and thoughts, you should try playing track 1 to get your mind a little more settled before going onto track 5. The track will begin to take the mind down in to a deep delta sleep. This is known as dreamless sleep and is the most restful and recuperative type of sleep you can get. It will both nourish your mind and your body.

References

1.
Rana, Deepak, The Secret Power of Lists, 2010
Neepradaka Press

2.
Oster G (1973). Auditory beats in the brain. Sci. Am.
229 (4): 94–102

Hutchison, Michael M. (1986). Megabrain: new tools
and techniques for brain growth and mind expansion.
New York: W. Morrow.

Blauert, J. Spatial hearing - the psychophysics of
human sound localization; MIT Press; Cambridge,
Massachusetts (1983), ch. 2.4

Slatky, Harald (1992): Algorithms for direction
specific Processing of Sound Signals - the Realization
of a binaural Cocktail-Party-Processor-System,
Dissertation, Ruhr-University Bochum, ch. 3

Spitzer MW, Semple MN 1998. Transformation of
binaural response properties in the ascending auditory
pathway: influence of time-varying interaural phase
disparity,. J. Neurophysiol. 80 (6): 3062–76.

Thaut MH (2003). Neural basis of rhythmic timing networks in the human brain. Ann. N. Y. Acad. Sci. 999: 364–73. doi:10.1196/annals.1284.044. PMID 14681157.

Barr DF, Mullin TA, Herbert PS. (1977). Application of binaural beat phenomenon with aphasic patients. Arch Otolaryngol. 103 (4): 192–194.

Gerken GM, Moushegian G, Stillman RD, Rupert AL (1975). Human frequency-following responses to monaural and binaural stimuli. Electroencephalography and clinical neurophysiology 38 (4): 379–86. doi:10.1016/0013-4694(75)90262-X.

Lane JD, Kasian SJ, Owens JE, Marsh GR (1998). Binaural auditory beats affect vigilance performance and mood. Physiol. Behav. 63 (2): 249–52.

Beatty J, Greenberg A, Deibler WP, O'Hanlon JF (1974). Operant control of occipital theta rhythm affects performance in a radar monitoring task. Science 183 (127): 871–3. doi:10.1126/science.183.4127.871

Wahbeh H, Calabrese C, Zwickey H (2007). Binaural beat technology in humans: a pilot study to assess psychologic and physiologic effects. Journal of alternative and complementary medicine (New York, N.Y.) 13 (1): 25–32. doi:10.1089/acm.2006.6196

L. Hson Nilsson   and E. Hultman Scandinavian Journal of Clinical & Laboratory Investigation 1973, Vol. 32, No. 4, Pages 325-330, Liver Glycogen in Man - the Effect of Total Starvation or a Carbohydrate-Poor Diet Followed by Carbohydrate Refeeding

<u>3.</u>

Kerr,J.S. (1991). Driving without attention mode (DWAM): a formalisation of inattentive states while driving. In Gale, A.G. et al. (Eds.), Vision in Vehicles III (pp. 473–479). Amsterdam: elsevier.

Miles,W. (1929). Sleeping with the Eyes Open. Scientific American, 489–492, June.

Schachter, D. (1976). The hypnagogic state: a critical review of the literature. Psychological Bulletin, 83 (3), 452–481.

4.

You are what you eat: Channel 4 broadcasting, UK

5.

Liberman, G, Lavine, A, 2003 Rags to riches Iuniverse

6.

Johnson, A, Frequency of Meals, American Journal of Clinical Nutrition, Vol. 85, No. 4, 981-988, April 2007

7.

Courbasson, Rizea, and Weiskopf , (2008). Emotional Eating among Individuals with Concurrent Eating and Substance Use Disorders. Journal of Mental Dietz W. H.. Does hunger cause obesity?. Pediatrics 1995;95:766-767

Murphy J. M., Wehler C. A., Pagano M. E., Little M., Kleinman R. E., Jellinek M. S.. Relationship between hunger and psychosocial functioning in low-income American children. J. Am. Acad. Child Adolesc. Psychiatry 1998;37:163-170

8.

Atkins RC. Dr Atkins' New Diet Revolution. Avon Books. New York. p57. 2002

Yancy WS, Guyton JR, Bakst RP et al., A randomized controlled trial of a very low carbohydrate diet with nutritional supplements versus low fat low-calorie diet, Obesity Research, 1998;37:163-170

9.

Batmanghelidj, B, .Benefits of Water, B.SCIENCE WATCH (Science Times) of the New York Times, Tuesday, June 21, 1983

Science or attitude? Science in medicine simplified 2:1-4 , June 1991

Thomas E. McKone Human exposure to volatile organic compounds in household tap water: the indoor inhalation pathway Environ. Sci. Technol., 1987, 21 (12), pp 1194–120

Smith, Billy L.; Handley, Priscilla; Eldredge, Dee, Ann Sex differences in exercise motivation and body-image satisfaction among college students. Perceptual and Motor Skills. Vol 86(2), Apr 1998, 723-732

Medicine & Science in Sports & Exercise: January 2006 - Volume 38 - Issue 1 - pp 179-188 Applied Sciences: Psychobiology and Behavoural Strategies Teixeira,

Pedro, J, Exercise Motivation, Eating, and Body Image Variables as Predictors of Weight Control Health Education Research Advance Access originally published online on November 13, 2006

F.B. Gillison, Relationships among adolescents' weight perceptions, exercise goals, exercise motivation, quality of life and leisure-time exercise behaviour: a self-determination theory approach Health Education Research 2006 21(6):836-847; doi:10.1093/her/cyl139 2000

Donna J. Plonczynski, Measurement of motivation for exercise Health Education Research, Vol. 15, No. 6, 695-705, December

Audio CD discount

Purchase the audio CD at a substantial discount off
the retail price.

Simply scan a proof of purchase and email your details
to Neepradaka press: NP@mrdee.net

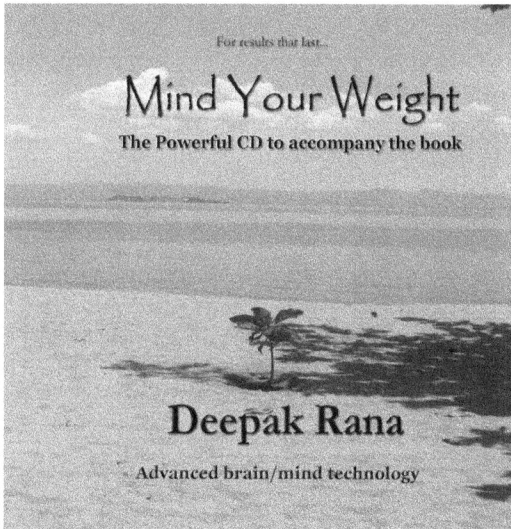

Index

To contact the author, or to keep up to date with new book releases email the publishers at:

NP@mrdee.net
www.np.mrdee.net

www.ingramcontent.com/pod-product-compliance
Lightning Source LLC
Chambersburg PA
CBHW050127280326
41933CB00010B/1284